Yoga

For Conception

Fertility Guide after PCOS/PCOD

Gabriel Wilson

Copyright © 2023 by Gabriel Wilson

ACKNOWLEDGEMENT

I want to express our sincerest gratitude and heartfelt gratitude to everyone who has selected this fertility guide as a companion on your road toward conception, especially as you traverse the unique hurdles provided by PCOS/PCOD.

Acceptance is a moment to celebrate the remarkable courage and perseverance that you bring to your pursuit of parenthood. The journey to becoming a parent can be a meandering one, with its share of challenges and uncertainty. Yet, you have made the daring choice to embrace yoga as a guiding light on this journey.

Living with PCOS/PCOD can pose its own set of difficulties, but your unshakeable resolve shows clearly as you investigate holistic approaches to increase your general health and fertility. Your commitment to these routines demonstrates a deep dedication to both your well-being and your desire for parenthood.

This guide is our way of expressing my appreciation and offering help. Within its pages, you'll find a wealth of knowledge, encouragement, and inspiration geared at strengthening you on your quest. We appreciate the unique nature of your journey, realizing that it can be a rollercoaster of emotions and problems.

While yoga can be an effective tool to improve your overall health and potentially enhance your fertility, it's crucial to stress the necessity of consulting with healthcare specialists who can provide specialized guidance targeted to your specific circumstances. Your path to motherhood is a comprehensive journey that may incorporate medical guidance, lifestyle adjustments, and the caring practice of yoga.

As you go forth on this path, please always remember that you are not alone. There is a community of support, and we are right here with you, every step of the way. Your tenacity, determination, and devotion to your well-being are tremendously inspiring. Together, we walk on with optimism, positivity, and the united conviction that brighter days await.

With heartfelt gratitude and kindest wishes,

GABRIEL WILSON

Allow me to introduce myself as a passionate advocate for natural health and yoga as a way to help people on their route to conception, especially those dealing with the challenges of PCOS/PCOD.

Gabriel Wilson offers this book with a lot of expertise and understanding. Gabriel Wilson, a committed yoga teacher with 12 years of experience, has seen the transformational effect of yoga on the mind, body, and spirit. He has witnessed how yoga may provide comfort and hope to those who are struggling with infertility.

Gabriel Wilson's path, however, goes beyond the yoga mat. He has dug deeply into the field of holistic longevity, realizing that genuine fertility includes not only the bodily but also the mental and spiritual parts of oneself. This handbook is a tribute to Gabriel Wilson's devotion to sharing this comprehensive knowledge with you, serving as a light of support and empowerment.

Thank you for entrusting Gabriel Wilson with your journey; he looks forward to accompanying you on your route to conception, health, and happiness.

Table of Contents

ACKNOWLEDGEMENT......................2

ABOUT THE AUTHOR......................6

INTRODUCTION 9

CHAPTER 1: UNDERSTANDING PCOS/PCOD AND FERTILITY CHALLENGES 17

CHAPTER 2: THE SCIENCE BEHIND YOGA AND FERTILITY ENHANCEMENT 37

CHAPTER 3: PREPARING THE MIND AND BODY FOR CONCEPTION 67

CHAPTER 4: YOGA PRACTICES FOR FERTILITY ENHANCEMENT 97

CHAPTER 5: DESIGNING A PERSONALIZED YOGA PRACTICE AND LIFESTYLE PLAN 157

INTRODUCTION

In the joyful embrace of life's twists and turns, our journey took us down a route we had never expected, one that unfurled into a narrative of perseverance, love, and the transformational power of yoga. Meet our family, where hope took the shape of a fertility guide after facing the hurdles of PCOS and PCOD and where the ancient practice of yoga became our guiding light toward conception.

In the core of our tale is the irrepressible spirit of my wife, Reye. Her fight with polycystic ovarian Syndrome (PCOS) had taxed her strength and dedication, but it couldn't destroy her spirit. With unshakable bravery, she weathered the emotional rollercoaster that typically accompanies reproductive issues. Amidst doctor's visits, therapies, and periods of doubt, she hung onto a dream to foster a new life inside her.

As we dug further into our search for conception, we noticed a novel emphasis on yoga for fertility. Drawn by the whispers of its therapeutic potential, we went on a quest to understand and harness the power of this ancient practice. Guided by professionals and armed with information, we began implementing particular yoga asana and breathing methods that were customized to meet the issues presented by PCOS But this voyage was not a lonely one. Our family, an unbreakable one, stood by each other's side. Together, we found consolation in the soothing beat of yoga. As the sun rose, we would meet on our yoga mats, ready to welcome the day with fresh energy. Breathing in rhythm, we connected with the cosmos, gathering power from the inside. It wasn't simply a physical workout; it was a spiritual and emotional tie that kept us together.

And as the weeks grew into months, we started to notice the subtle modifications not only in our bodies but in our hearts and minds. The tension that had previously threaded its way into our lives started to weaken its hold. The daily practice of yoga, mixed with the warmth of togetherness, injected a feeling of tranquility that we had been seeking. It seemed as if we were sowing seeds of optimism, caring for them with every attentive breath and stretch.

With time, the transformational impact of yoga became clear. The asana meant to stimulate the reproductive system, along with the concentration on mindfulness, were beginning to yield promising outcomes. But beyond the outward changes, something deeper was at play: a newfound connection with our bodies and a profound comprehension of the delicate dance of life inside.

Our experience is a testimony to the reality that the road to conception is filled with more than just medical procedures it's a comprehensive route that demands nourishing the body, mind, and soul. As our family's journey continues to unfold, we carry with us the knowledge of yoga and the strong link that it has built. It's a narrative of hope, resilience, and the tremendous power that resides within us when we open ourselves to the transforming path of yoga.

Welcome to the entire guide on Yoga for Conception: Fertility after PCOS/PCOD. Embarking on the journey towards conception may be both exhilarating and hard, particularly for individuals who have experienced challenges such as Polycystic Ovary Syndrome (PCOS) or Polycystic Ovarian Disease (PCOD). These conditions may impair fertility, but the ancient practice of yoga provides a comprehensive approach to increasing fertility, promoting hormonal balance, and nourishing general well-being.

In this guide, we will dig into the remarkable synergy between yoga and fertility, geared particularly for people navigating the complications of PCOS/PCOD. We will examine how mindful movement, breath work, relaxation methods, and a caring mentality may balance the body and mind, possibly enhancing the odds of conception while reducing some of the obstacles caused by these conditions.

Whether you are new to yoga or have an experienced practice, this guide will give you insights, into yoga postures, sequences, and mindfulness practices that may assist in balancing hormones, lowering stress, boosting circulation, and creating an environment suitable for conception. Remember, this journey is unique to each person, and the objective is to equip you with skills that may be incorporated into your lifestyle, promoting a healthy and harmonious road to fertility.

From developing inner quiet to fostering a positive view of this chapter of your life, the activities inside this guide are meant to promote not just physical health but also emotional well-being. Embrace the knowledge of yoga as you traverse the road of conception, discovering balance, strength, and tranquility within yourself. Let's start on this transforming journey together, embracing the possibilities for fresh beginnings and the pleasures that lie ahead.

Chapter 1: Understanding PCOS/PCOD and Fertility Challenges

Polycystic Ovary Syndrome (PCOS), also known as Polycystic Ovary Disease (PCOD), is a common hormonal condition that affects people with ovaries, generally during their reproductive years. It is a complicated illness that may lead to different health difficulties, including reproductive challenges. Let's review PCOS/PCOD and its link to reproductive issues in greater depth.

Understanding PCOS/PCOD: PCOS is defined by a variety of symptoms, which may vary in severity across people. The specific etiology of PCOS is not entirely known, but it includes a hormonal imbalance, including high levels of androgens (male hormones), insulin resistance, and an irregular menstrual cycle.

Common signs of PCOS/PCOD include:

Irregular Menstrual Cycles: Women with PCOS may have infrequent or protracted menstrual cycles, or they could suffer irregular periods.

Ovulatory Dysfunction: Ovulation may be irregular or nonexistent in people with PCOS, leading to difficulties in conceiving.

Hyperandrogenism: Elevated androgen levels may contribute to symptoms including acne, abundant facial and body hair (hirsutism), and male-pattern baldness.

Polycystic Ovaries: Despite the term, not all patients with PCOS have cysts on their ovaries. However, individuals may have several tiny cyst-like follicles on their ovaries when seen by ultrasonography.

Insulin Resistance: Insulin resistance is frequent in PCOS and may lead to weight gain and problems maintaining blood sugar levels.

Fertility Challenges: One of the biggest concerns for those with PCOS is the effect it may have on fertility. The irregular ovulation or absence of ovulation might make it difficult to conceive naturally. When ovulation doesn't occur consistently, the chances of fertilization and pregnancy are lowered.

However, it's crucial to understand that not all persons with PCOS may encounter reproductive troubles. Some could have little problem conceiving, while others may need medical help. **Treatments for PCOS-related reproductive difficulties include:**

Lifestyle Modifications: Maintaining a healthy weight via food and exercise may assist in improving hormonal balance and enhance the chance of regular ovulation.

Drugs: Hormonal drugs such as clomiphene citrate or letrozole may be recommended to stimulate ovulation.

Assisted Reproductive methods (ART): In more severe instances of PCOS-related infertility, methods including in vitro fertilization (IVF) or intrauterine insemination (IUI) might be employed.

Ovulation Induction: Hormonal injections may induce ovulation in persons with PCOS.

Management of Insulin Resistance: If insulin resistance is a substantial problem, medicines to increase insulin sensitivity may be recommended.

PCOS/PCOD is a complicated hormonal condition that may have a considerable influence on fertility owing to irregular ovulation or anovulation. While it might offer obstacles, many people with PCOS can conceive with the correct therapies and support. If you believe you have PCOS and are having reproductive challenges, it's vital to speak with a medical specialist who can give the correct diagnosis and assistance customized to your unique circumstances.

Impact of PCOS/PCOD on Fertility

Polycystic Ovary Syndrome (PCOS) and Polycystic Ovary Disease (PCOD) are prevalent endocrine illnesses that impact the reproductive health of humans, especially women. While the names are commonly used interchangeably, PCOS is more generally known and utilized. PCOS/PCOD may have a substantial influence on fertility owing to the hormonal abnormalities and accompanying symptoms it produces. **Here's a debate about the influence of PCOS/PCOD on fertility:**

Anovulation: One of the principal implications of PCOS on fertility is anovulation, which means the ovaries do not produce eggs consistently. Normally, a developed egg is delivered from the ovaries throughout each menstrual cycle, allowing for fertilization. In women with PCOS, hormonal abnormalities disturb this process, resulting in irregular or missing ovulation. This drastically diminishes the odds of conception.

Hormonal Imbalances: PCOS is characterized by high amounts of androgens (male hormones) such as testosterone, as well as insulin resistance. These hormonal abnormalities may interfere with the normal ovulation process and can affect the formation of ovarian follicles, which are important for egg maturation.

Menstrual Irregularities: Irregular or nonexistent menstrual cycles are frequent in women with PCOS. This is commonly a consequence of anovulation and hormone abnormalities. Irregular cycles might make it difficult to anticipate the fertile window, making it tougher to schedule intercourse for conception.

Ovarian Cysts: While not all women with PCOS have ovarian cysts, the word itself indicates the presence of many tiny cysts on the ovaries. These cysts are follicles that have not developed adequately owing to hormonal abnormalities. Their presence might further lead to irregular ovulation and reproductive difficulties.

Impact on Egg Quality: Even when ovulation does occur in women with PCOS, the quality of the eggs produced may be affected. This may disrupt fertilization and embryo development, leading to an increased chance of miscarriage.

Increased chance of Miscarriage: Women with PCOS have a greater chance of miscarriage compared to those without the disease. The causes for this are complicated and likely involve variables such as hormone imbalances, irregular ovulation, and probable concerns with egg quality.

Lifestyle Factors: Insulin resistance is typically associated with PCOS. Insulin resistance may lead to obesity and other metabolic disorders. These variables may further contribute to reproductive issues since obesity itself is connected with lower fertility.

Medicinal Intervention: Many women with PCOS need medicinal intervention to assist in controlling their menstrual periods and stimulate ovulation. Fertility treatments such as ovulation-inducing medicines (e.g., Clomid) or assisted reproductive technologies like in vitro fertilization (IVF) may be prescribed for people struggling to conceive.

Long-Term Health consequences: Beyond fertility, PCOS/PCOD may have significant health consequences such as a higher risk of type 2 diabetes, cardiovascular disease, and endometrial cancer. Managing the illness with lifestyle modifications, medication, and frequent medical check-ups is vital for general health and reproductive well-being.

It's crucial to remember that the influence of PCOS/PCOD on fertility differs from person to person. While some people could encounter considerable difficulty, others might have less severe reproductive concerns. If you feel you have PCOS and are dealing with fertility, it's essential to seek medical counsel. A healthcare expert may give a tailored evaluation and propose suitable therapies to boost your chances of conception.

Common Fertility Challenges Associate with PCOS/PCOD

Polycystic Ovary Syndrome (PCOS), also known as Polycystic Ovary Disease (PCOD), is a hormonal condition that affects persons with ovaries, especially during their reproductive years. One of the biggest concerns connected with PCOS/PCOD is reproductive issues. Let's explore the typical reproductive issues connected with PCOS/PCOD:

Anovulation: Anovulation refers to the absence of ovulation or irregular ovulation, which is a characteristic of PCOS/PCOD. Ovulation is necessary for successful conception because it releases an egg that can be fertilized by sperm. In PCOS/PCOD, hormonal abnormalities disturb the typical ovulatory cycle, making it difficult to anticipate when ovulation will occur.

Irregular Menstrual Cycles: PCOS/PCOD commonly leads to irregular menstrual cycles, characterized by unexpected or infrequent periods. This inconsistency might make it tough to predict the viable window for conception since the cycle duration differs from person to person.

Hormonal Imbalances: PCOS/PCOD is characterized by high levels of androgens (male hormones) such as testosterone, as well as insulin resistance. These hormonal abnormalities may interfere with the growth and release of mature eggs from the ovaries.

Ovulatory Dysfunction: Even when ovulation occurs in persons with PCOS/PCOD, the quality of ovulation might be reduced. The eggs released can be of lesser quality, lowering the odds of successful fertilization and implantation.

High LH-to-FSH Ratio: In a normal menstrual cycle, luteinizing hormone (LH) and follicle-stimulating hormone (FSH) are produced in particular ratios. In PCOS/PCOD, the ratio is commonly disturbed, resulting in excessive levels of LH. This may lead to the production of ovarian cysts and inhibit ovulation.

Ovarian Cysts: Follicles that fail to mature into eggs might develop into ovarian cysts. These cysts may collect and develop over time, leading to hormonal imbalances and further interfering with regular ovulation.

Endometrial Abnormalities: Hormonal imbalances in PCOS/PCOD may lead to abnormalities in the uterine lining (endometrium), making it difficult for a fertilized egg to implant and mature normally.

Insulin Resistance: Many patients with PCOS/PCOD also develop insulin resistance, a condition where the body's cells do not react adequately to insulin. This may lead to greater amounts of insulin in the blood, which in turn can alter ovarian function and contribute to infertility.

Obesity: While not all patients with PCOS/PCOD are overweight, obesity is a prevalent issue. Excess weight may increase hormonal imbalances and insulin resistance, further impacting fertility.

Factors: Unhealthy lifestyle behaviors, such as poor food, lack of exercise, and excessive stress, may increase the symptoms of PCOS/PCOD and lead to reproductive issues.

fertility issues linked with PCOS/PCOD frequently need a mix of medical therapies, lifestyle adjustments, and assisted reproductive technology. Treatments could include drugs to stimulate ovulation, lifestyle adjustments to increase insulin sensitivity, weight management, and in vitro fertilization (IVF) in more severe instances.

If you're suffering fertility troubles due to PCOS/PCOD, it's crucial to contact a healthcare professional or a reproductive endocrinologist who specializes in fertility concerns. They may give unique assistance and suggestions depending on your scenario.

The Role of Lifestyle Factors in Conception

Lifestyle variables have a key effect on conception and fertility for both men and women. These variables may impact the likelihood of successful conception by altering hormonal balance, reproductive health, and general well-being. Here's a discussion of several significant lifestyle elements that affect conception:

Nutrition and Diet: A balanced and healthy diet is vital for reproductive health. Nutrient deficiencies, such as folic acid, zinc, and vitamin D, might impair fertility. Excessive use of processed meals, trans fats, and sugary goods may lead to hormonal abnormalities and obesity, which may significantly affect fertility.

Body Weight: Both underweight and overweight disorders might contribute to reproductive issues. Obesity may affect hormonal balance, resulting in irregular menstrual periods and diminished ovulation. Conversely, too thinness may contribute to irregular periods and anovulation (lack of ovulation).

Exercise and Physical Activity: Regular moderate exercise is typically excellent for fertility and overall health. However, overly intense activity in women might lead to irregular periods and disturbed ovulation. Finding a balance between physical exercise and reproductive health is vital.

Smoking: Smoking, as well as exposure to secondhand smoke, has been associated with lower fertility in both men and women. It may adversely influence sperm quality, hormone production, and egg quality.

Alcohol use: Excessive alcohol use has been connected with lower fertility in both men and women. It may alter hormonal balance and damage sperm and egg quality.

Caffeine Intake: While moderate caffeine intake is typically regarded safe, large amounts of caffeine consumption may impact fertility in certain women. It's suggested to minimize caffeine consumption, particularly during the preconception period.

Stress: Chronic stress may lead to hormonal abnormalities that impair the reproductive system. Stress reduction practices, including meditation, yoga, and relaxation exercises, may promote conception.

Sleep Patterns: Irregular sleep patterns and severe sleep deprivation might affect hormone balance and impair fertility. Prioritizing excellent sleep hygiene is vital for general health and reproductive well-being.

Environmental Toxins: Exposure to environmental toxins, such as pesticides, pollution, and some chemicals, may impair fertility in both men and women. Minimizing exposure to these poisons is advised.

Age: While not a lifestyle component per se, age plays a vital influence on fertility. Fertility falls with age, particularly in women, owing to a reduction in the amount and quality of eggs. It's crucial to be mindful of the biological clock while preparing for conception.

Sexual Health: Maintaining excellent sexual health, including addressing concerns like sexually transmitted infections (STIs), is vital for overall reproductive well-being.

It's worth mentioning that the influence of lifestyle variables on conception might differ from person to person. Making healthy lifestyle adjustments long in advance of attempting to conceive may dramatically boost the odds of a successful pregnancy.

Chapter 2: The Science Behind Yoga and Fertility Enhancement

The possible association between yoga and fertility improvement is an area of research that has attracted attention in recent years. While there isn't a solid scientific agreement on the specific processes via which yoga could directly promote fertility, various characteristics connected with yoga practice might lead to enhanced reproductive results. It's crucial to highlight that although some studies imply good impacts, additional study is required to establish clear causal relationships.

Here are several ways in which yoga might impact fertility:

Stress Reduction: Yoga generally combines deep breathing, relaxation methods, and mindfulness practices, which may help decrease stress and promote relaxation. High amounts of stress may severely disrupt reproductive hormones and menstrual cycles, possibly impacting fertility. By controlling stress, yoga may indirectly assist greater reproductive health.

Hormonal Balance: Certain yoga postures and practices are considered to stimulate and massage the endocrine system, which plays a critical role in controlling hormones. Balancing hormones including cortisol, thyroid hormones, and reproductive hormones like estrogen and progesterone may lead to better menstrual cycles and enhanced fertility.

Blood Circulation: Yoga poses frequently include moderate stretching and movement that may increase blood circulation throughout the body. This enhanced circulation may aid the reproductive organs by delivering a healthy supply of oxygen and nutrients, which can boost their performance.

Pelvic Floor Health: Yoga contains activities that target the muscles of the pelvic floor. Strengthening the pelvic floor muscles may have significant impacts on reproductive health by possibly enhancing blood flow to the reproductive organs and promoting overall pelvic health.

Body Weight Regulation: Maintaining a healthy body weight is vital for fertility. Certain yoga practices may aid with weight control by developing mindful eating habits, greater physical activity, and a stronger connection between the mind and body.

Neuroendocrine Effects: Yoga's effect on the neurological system may alter the release of hormones that govern many biological activities, including reproduction. Practices like meditation and relaxation methods could indirectly alter the hypothalamus and pituitary glands, which are essential actors in the reproductive hormone cascade.

Improved Lifestyle Choices: Engaging in yoga frequently goes hand-in-hand with adopting a healthy lifestyle, including a balanced diet, regular exercise, and less usage of dangerous drugs. These lifestyle modifications may significantly benefit general health, including reproductive health.

While there is some early research showing that yoga could have good impacts on fertility, it's vital to view these statements with care. Scientific research in this field is still beginning, and more rigorous studies are required to demonstrate definite cause-and-effect correlations between yoga and fertility improvement. If you're contemplating yoga as part of your fertility journey, it's a good idea to talk with medical specialists and fertility experts to establish the most effective method for your unique circumstances.

How Yoga Affects the Body and Mind

Yoga is a comprehensive discipline that has been around for thousands of years and is recognized for its therapeutic benefits on both the body and the mind. It blends physical postures, breathing methods, meditation, and ethical ideals to enhance general well-being. The effects of yoga on the body and mind are interrelated and may be extremely deep.

Effects on the Body:

Flexibility and Strength: Yoga incorporates some positions and stretches that focus on various muscle groups. Over time, these activities build flexibility and enhance muscular strength. This may lead to improved posture, a lower chance of accidents, and increased body awareness.

Balance and Coordination: Many yoga postures demand balance and coordination, which serve to develop proprioception (awareness of body position) and stability. This may be particularly effective for elderly persons in avoiding falls.

Stress Reduction: Practicing yoga affects the parasympathetic nervous system, promoting the relaxation response. This leads to lower levels of stress chemicals like cortisol, which in turn may have a good influence on numerous biological systems.

Cardiovascular Health: Certain styles of yoga, such as Vinyasa or Power Yoga, may give cardiovascular exercise by boosting the heart rate. This may assist in enhancing circulation, heart health, and general stamina.

Pain Management: Yoga has been proven to reduce numerous forms of pain, including back pain, arthritis, and migraines. The combination of stretching, strengthening, and relaxation practices may aid in pain reduction.

Respiratory Health: Yoga emphasizes regulated breathing (pranayama), which helps increase lung capacity and respiratory function. This is especially good for persons with respiratory disorders like asthma.

Benefits on the Mind:

Tension and Anxiety Reduction: One of the most well-known benefits of yoga is its ability to relieve tension and anxiety. Mindfulness practices employed in yoga, such as deep breathing and meditation, help settle the mind and generate a feeling of calmness.

Attention and Awareness: Yoga increases present-moment awareness and attention. Practicing mindfulness on the mat typically transfers into enhanced awareness in everyday life, promoting a stronger appreciation of the present moment.

Mental Clarity and Focus: Regular yoga practice has been related to increased cognitive function, including greater focus and mental clarity. The combination of physical exercise and conscious awareness may help eliminate mental clutter.

Emotional Regulation: Yoga may help people control their emotions by improving emotional awareness and regulation. It gives a safe area to examine and process emotions that may be held in the body.

Self-Reflection and Self-Discovery: The contemplative features of yoga stimulate introspection and self-discovery. This may lead to a greater knowledge of oneself, one's values, and life's purpose.

Positive view: Yoga philosophy generally emphasizes positive attitudes and ethical ideals, which may lead to a more optimistic view of life and enhanced interpersonal interactions.

In summary, yoga is a multifaceted practice that impacts both the body and mind in different ways. Its physical advantages include greater flexibility, strength, and balance, while its mental benefits involve stress reduction, enhanced mindfulness, and emotional well-being. The interconnection of these impacts makes yoga a holistic approach to general health and wellbeing.

Yoga's Impact on Hormonal Balance

Yoga is a comprehensive discipline that involves physical postures, breathing exercises, meditation, and ethical ideals. While there is minimal empirical scientific study explicitly focused on the influence of yoga on hormone balance, there is evidence to indicate that practicing yoga may have favorable benefits on several hormonal systems inside the body. These impacts may contribute to overall hormonal balance and well-being.

Here's how yoga could affect hormone balance:

Stress Reduction: One of the most well-documented advantages of yoga is its ability to relieve stress. Chronic stress may lead to an imbalance in hormones such as cortisol, adrenaline, and norepinephrine. Regular yoga practice has been found to stimulate the parasympathetic nervous system, prompting the relaxation response. This, in turn, may help lower the body's stress hormone levels and improve hormonal stability.

Endocrine System Regulation: The endocrine system is responsible for creating and regulating hormones. Certain yoga postures and practices may stimulate certain glands within the endocrine system, possibly aiding their optimum functioning. For example, inverted positions like shoulder stand and headstand are considered to impact the thyroid gland, which plays a critical role in controlling metabolism and energy balance.

Blood Sugar Regulation: Some research shows that yoga could help manage blood sugar levels. This might be advantageous for persons with problems like insulin resistance or diabetes. By favorably affecting blood sugar regulation, yoga could indirectly regulate hormones associated with metabolism and energy management.

Hormones and Mood: Yoga has been related to benefits in mood and mental well-being. Practicing yoga may boost the production of "feel-good" chemicals such as endorphins and serotonin, while concurrently lowering the levels of stress hormones. This exchange may help to emotional equilibrium and a happy attitude.

Hormones and Reproductive Health: Certain yoga practices, such as restorative positions and deep breathing exercises, may help regulate the menstrual cycle and ease symptoms of disorders including polycystic ovarian syndrome (PCOS) and premenstrual syndrome (PMS). Yoga's stress-reducing benefits may also indirectly alter reproductive hormone balance.

Cortisol Regulation: Cortisol, frequently referred to as the "stress hormone," plays a critical function in the body's reaction to stress. Chronic increased cortisol levels might have detrimental impacts on health. Regular yoga practice has been related to decreased cortisol levels, which may produce a more balanced hormonal state.

Mind-Body Connection: Yoga promotes the mind-body connection and awareness of physical sensations. This heightened awareness may lead to improved identification of hormone imbalances and their impact on the body. By listening to these cues, people may be more proactive in seeking appropriate medical measures if required.

It's crucial to remember that individual reactions to yoga might vary, and the influence on hormone balance might not be the same for everyone. While yoga may be a beneficial supplemental exercise for achieving hormonal balance, it should not replace conventional medical therapy. If you want to treat particular hormonal disorders, it's essential to talk with healthcare specialists who specialize in endocrinology and consider incorporating yoga into a holistic wellness plan.

Stress Reduction and Fertility

Stress may have a substantial influence on several elements of our physical and emotional well-being, including fertility. While the link between stress and fertility is complicated and not completely understood, there is evidence to indicate that excessive levels of stress might impair reproductive health. Here's how stress reduction and fertility are interconnected:

Hormonal Imbalance: Stress promotes the production of chemicals like cortisol and adrenaline, which are part of the body's "fight or flight" response. Prolonged exposure to these stress hormones may disturb the balance of other hormones that are necessary for reproductive function, such as those involved in regulating the menstrual cycle and ovulation in women and sperm generation in men.

Menstrual Irregularities: High levels of stress may lead to irregular menstrual periods or even amenorrhea (lack of menstruation). These changes in the menstrual cycle might make it more complicated for women to anticipate ovulation and conceive.

Ovulation: Stress may influence the secretion of luteinizing hormone (LH) and follicle-stimulating hormone (FSH), which are crucial for inducing ovulation. In certain circumstances, stress-related hormonal alterations might result in anovulation (lack of ovulation), making conception problematic.

Sperm Quality: subjected to prolonged stress may see changes in sperm quality and quantity. Stress may alter testosterone levels and sperm production, possibly leading to lower sperm count and motility.

Psychological Factors: The emotional toll of infertility itself may add to stress and anxiety. The fertility journey may be emotionally exhausting, leading to a loop where stress impacts fertility and reproductive concerns and, in turn, generates additional stress.

Given these probable linkages, stress reduction techniques may play a role in boosting fertility:

Mind-Body Techniques: Practices like meditation, deep breathing, and yoga have been demonstrated to lower stress levels and increase relaxation. These strategies may help control stress hormones and create a more favorable atmosphere for reproductive health.

Counseling and Support: Seeking emotional support via counseling, support groups, or talking to a therapist may help individuals and couples with coping tools to handle the stress associated with reproductive issues.

Physical Activity: Regular exercise may help relieve stress and increase general well-being. However, excessive and vigorous exercise could also have detrimental effects on fertility, so balance is crucial.

Healthy Lifestyle: A balanced diet, enough sleep, and avoiding excessive alcohol and caffeine consumption might lead to both stress reduction and enhanced fertility.

Mindfulness and Relaxation: Engaging in mindfulness activities might help people handle stress and anxiety more efficiently, possibly benefitting their reproductive health.

Communication: Openly discussing with a spouse about reproductive difficulties and seeking mutual support may help reduce some of the emotional load.

It's crucial to remember that although stress reduction measures might be beneficial, they might not address underlying medical issues influencing fertility. Individuals and couples coping with fertility concerns should visit medical specialists who specialize in reproductive health to obtain thorough counseling and suitable solutions.

Enhancing Blood Circulation to Reproductive Organs through Yoga

Enhancing blood circulation to reproductive organs is considered to offer several advantages for both men and women, including increased sexual health, fertility, and general reproductive function. Yoga, a comprehensive practice that incorporates physical postures, breathing techniques, meditation, and awareness, has been recommended as a possible strategy to boost blood circulation to the reproductive organs. While scientific data on the direct benefits of yoga on reproductive organ circulation is still evolving, there are various avenues via which yoga might contribute to enhanced circulation in these regions.

Physical Movement and Poses (Asanas): Yoga incorporates a sequence of physical postures that stretch and flex specific muscle groups. Certain yoga positions may especially target the pelvic area, which contains the reproductive organs. Poses like the Butterfly Pose

(Baddha Konasana), Pigeon Pose (Eka Pada Rajakapotasana), and Wide-Legged Forward Bend (Prasarita Padottanasana) might assist in loosening up the hips and enhance blood flow to the pelvic region.

Deep Breathing methods (Pranayama): Pranayama comprises regulated and deep breathing methods. These treatments are supposed to increase oxygen flow to the body's cells and tissues, including the reproductive organs. Improved oxygenation may enhance overall organ function, perhaps including greater blood circulation to certain locations.

Relaxation and Stress Reduction: Chronic stress may significantly affect blood circulation throughout the body, particularly to the reproductive organs. Yoga's focus on relaxation, mindfulness, and meditation may help decrease stress and maintain a healthy blood flow by reducing constriction of blood vessels owing to stress-induced reactions.

Activation of the Parasympathetic Nervous System: Yoga activities generally activate the parasympathetic nervous system, which is responsible for the "rest and digest" response. This activation may lead to vasodilation (relaxation of blood vessels), facilitating enhanced blood circulation throughout the body.

Improved Flexibility and Blood Flow: Regular yoga practice may enhance general flexibility and muscular tone. This may assist in maintaining appropriate posture, minimizing muscular imbalances, and ensuring that blood vessels are not constricted owing to strained muscles.

Increased Core Strength: Many yoga postures require the use of the core muscles. A strong core may aid in maintaining proper posture and supporting the spine, which in turn can contribute to enhanced blood circulation to the lower abdomen and pelvic area.

While there is anecdotal evidence showing that yoga may favorably improve reproductive health, more rigorous scientific study is required to demonstrate a definite cause-and-effect link between yoga and better blood circulation to reproductive organs. If you're interested in utilizing yoga to boost reproductive health, it's crucial to check with healthcare specialists, such as gynecologists or urologists, particularly if you have any pre-existing issues or concerns.

Remember that yoga is usually regarded as safe for most people, but it's crucial to practice under the instruction of a competent yoga teacher, especially if you're new to yoga. Additionally, integrating yoga with a balanced diet, frequent exercise, and a healthy lifestyle may help to overall reproductive health and well-being.

Chapter 3: Preparing the Mind and Body for Conception

Preparing the mind and body for conception is a comprehensive approach to boosting the odds of a healthy pregnancy. It entails making lifestyle changes, adopting healthy behaviors, and treating psychological problems to provide an ideal environment for conception to occur. This procedure is crucial for both couples since the general health and well-being of both the mother and the father might affect fertility and the health of the future child.

Here are some crucial factors in preparing the mind and body for conception:

Healthy Diet: A balanced and healthy diet is vital for fertility. Consuming a mix of fruits, vegetables, whole grains, lean proteins, and healthy fats offers critical nutrients that promote reproductive health. Nutrients including folic acid, zinc, iron, and antioxidants have a role in fertility.

Maintaining a Healthy Weight: Both underweight and overweight situations may adversely influence fertility. Maintaining a healthy weight via regular exercise and a balanced diet might enhance hormonal balance and boost the chances of conception.

Regular Exercise: Engaging in regular physical exercise not only helps maintain a healthy weight but also promotes blood circulation and general well-being. However, excessive activity or severe fitness programs may occasionally adversely affect fertility, so balance is crucial.

Managing Stress: High levels of stress might disturb hormonal balance and ovulation. Practicing stress-reduction practices like meditation, yoga, deep breathing, and mindfulness may increase relaxation and favorably enhance fertility.

Adequate Sleep: Getting adequate restful sleep is vital for hormone control and general wellness. Sleep deprivation may lead to hormonal changes that could impact fertility.

Avoiding Harmful Substances: Both couples should avoid substances including cigarettes, alcohol, recreational drugs, and excessive coffee, since they might impact fertility and raise the chance of pregnancy difficulties.

Regular Health Checkups: Before trying conception, it's essential to undergo a full medical examination to treat any underlying health concerns or diseases that can influence fertility. This includes treating chronic conditions and ensuring vaccines are up to date.

Timing Intercourse: Understanding the menstrual cycle and recognizing the fertile window (when ovulation occurs) is critical for successful conception.

Tracking basal body temperature, and cervical mucus changes, and utilizing ovulation prediction kits may assist in pinpointing the optimal time for intercourse.

Open Communication: Both parties must discuss honestly their thoughts, fears, and expectations surrounding conception and motherhood. This develops emotional support and minimizes stress.

Supporting Emotional Health: Dealing with infertility may be emotionally taxing. Seeking help from friends, family, or a mental health professional may be effective in handling these feelings.

Prenatal Care: Once conception occurs, early prenatal care is critical for a healthy pregnancy. This involves taking prenatal vitamins, having frequent checkups, and following medical instructions.

Remember that the route to conception may differ for each person or couple, and there's no one-size-fits-all strategy. Consulting with healthcare experts, such as obstetricians, gynecologists, and fertility specialists, may give individualized recommendations based on particular circumstances.

Cultivating a Positive Mindset for Fertility

Cultivating a good mentality for fertility requires adopting a psychological and emotional approach that helps your path toward conception and family-building. While a happy outlook doesn't ensure reproductive success, it may add to your general well-being and perhaps improve your fertility-related experiences. Here's how you can focus on creating a good mentality for fertility:

Acknowledge and Manage Stress: High stress levels may severely affect fertility. Cultivating a happy mentality entails understanding the causes of stress and finding appropriate strategies to handle them. Practices like meditation, yoga, deep breathing, and mindfulness may help decrease stress and improve emotional balance.

Focus on Self-Care: Prioritize self-care activities that improve physical, mental, and emotional well-being. This can involve indulging in activities you like, spending time with loved ones, getting appropriate sleep, and keeping a healthy diet. Taking care of your whole health might significantly affect your reproductive journey.

Practice hope: While it's vital to be realistic about the problems you encounter, keeping a feeling of hope might make the path less emotionally exhausting. Focus on positive areas of your life, set reasonable objectives, and remind yourself of your strengths and perseverance.

Avoid Negative Self-Talk: Negative self-talk may weaken your self-confidence and add to thoughts of despair. Challenge and reframe negative beliefs that could develop throughout your reproductive journey. Replace them with more positive and constructive self-affirmations.

Seek Support: Connect with people who are on a similar path or seek out specialists who specialize in fertility and reproductive health. Joining support groups or seeking counseling may offer you a secure environment to discuss your thoughts and gain insights into handling the emotional side of reproductive issues.

Set Realistic Expectations: Fertility may be unexpected, and setbacks are normal. Cultivating a good mentality entails realizing that the trip could have ups and downs. Setting reasonable expectations might help you handle disappointment while retaining a cheerful attitude.

Visualize Success: Visualizing optimistic results may profoundly influence your thinking. Consider using strategies like visualization or making vision boards that illustrate your intended family-building path. These tools might act as reminders of your aims and desires.

Maintain Open Communication: Keep the lines of communication open with your spouse. Sharing your thoughts, concerns, and hopes may improve your relationship and help you manage obstacles together.

Practice gratitude: Focusing on the good parts of your life and expressing thanks for what you have may transform your perspective and enhance your general well-being. Keeping a thankfulness book or even spending a minute each day to focus on what you're grateful for may make a difference.

Stay Informed but Balanced: Educating oneself about fertility choices and treatments is crucial, but be mindful not to overload yourself with knowledge. Maintain a good balance between remaining informed and avoiding information overload.

Remember that everyone's reproductive journey is unique, and what works for one person may not work for another. The purpose of building a positive mentality is to promote your emotional well-being and resilience while you navigate the difficulties and rewards of your reproductive journey.

Yoga and Mindfulness Techniques for Stress Management

Yoga and mindfulness methods are incredibly effective strategies for controlling stress and boosting general well-being. Both disciplines have ancient origins and provide a comprehensive approach to alleviating stress by blending physical postures, breath control, meditation, and self-awareness. Let's look into each of these techniques and how they help with stress management:

Yoga:

Yoga is a holistic technique that integrates physical postures (asanas), breath control (pranayama), meditation, and ethical concepts to build a healthy mind and body. It's not just about flexibility or physical exercise; it's a comprehensive approach to obtaining mental and emotional harmony.

Physical Asanas: Yoga poses help alleviate physical stress, develop flexibility, and improve circulation. The practice of asanas may produce a feeling of achievement and relaxation, counteracting the physical consequences of stress.

Breath Control (Pranayama): Pranayama includes breath control methods that may have a direct influence on the neurological system. Practices like deep breathing, alternative nostril breathing, and soothing breathing help stimulate the body's relaxation response, lowering tension and anxiety.

Meditation: Yoga contains many meditation practices that foster attention and present-moment awareness. Mindful meditation, concentration methods (such as concentrating on a mantra), and guided imagery may assist in regulating racing thoughts and generating a feeling of calm.

Mind-Body Connection: Yoga stresses the link between the mind and body. Through mindful movement, people may become more attentive to their bodily experiences, fostering self-awareness and self-care.

Mindfulness:

Mindfulness is the discipline of devoting non-judgmental attention to the present moment. It entails growing awareness of ideas, emotions, physiological sensations, and the surrounding environment. Mindfulness-based stress reduction (MBSR) and mindfulness-based cognitive therapy (MBCT) are two well-known mindfulness methods.

Mindful Awareness: Mindfulness practices promote monitoring thoughts and emotions without judgment. This may lessen the harmful effect of stress by avoiding automatic reactions and allowing for more considered answers.

Body Scan: This mindfulness exercise includes mentally scanning your body to discover areas of tension, stress, or discomfort. The act of recognizing and accepting these feelings might enhance calm.

Breath Awareness: Focusing on the breath in the present moment helps anchor focus and produce a feeling of tranquility. It's a simple but effective technique to manage stress and maintain a concentrated state of mind.

Mindful Eating: Mindful eating involves giving full attention to the act of eating, enjoying each mouthful, and being mindful of the sensory experience. This may lead to improved eating habits and a decreased dependence on stress-induced eating.

Both yoga and mindfulness approaches may be tailored to individual tastes and requirements. Incorporating these activities into your daily routine may lead to long-term benefits in stress management, emotional control, and general well-being. It's vital to approach these routines with patience and regularity since the advantages tend to compound over time. If you're new to these techniques, consider obtaining advice from experienced teachers or resources to ensure you're practicing safely and successfully.

Balancing Emotional Well-being with Yoga

Balancing emotional well-being with yoga is a comprehensive strategy that integrates the physical practice of yoga with mindfulness, breathwork, and relaxation methods to enhance mental and emotional health. Yoga has been performed for hundreds of years and is recognized for its capacity to foster a feeling of inner calm, relieve stress, and increase general well-being.

Here's how yoga may assist to emotional balance:

Mind-Body Connection: Yoga stresses the link between the mind and body. Through mindful movement and body awareness, people may become more attentive to their emotions and physical sensations. This awareness assists in detecting emotional triggers and reacting to them in a balanced way.

Stress Reduction: Practicing yoga stimulates the parasympathetic nervous system, which promotes relaxation and lowers the "fight or flight" response associated with stress. As a consequence, stress chemicals like cortisol decrease, leading to a more steady and peaceful emotional state.

Mindfulness: Many styles of yoga involve mindfulness methods, urging practitioners to concentrate on the present moment without judgment. This technique may lead to a reduction in rumination, which is a major factor in anxiety and depression.

Breathwork (Pranayama): Yoga lays great emphasis on breath control. Pranayama methods include conscious regulation of the breath, which may have a direct influence on the autonomic nervous system. Deep, calm breathing helps stimulate the relaxation response, lowering anxiety and fostering emotional equilibrium.

Emotion Regulation: Yoga offers a safe and supportive place to explore and regulate emotions. The practice of holding positions and accepting physical pain may transfer to increased emotional resilience and tolerance of discomfort in everyday   life.

Relief Tension: Certain yoga positions assist in relieving physical tension held in the body. This tension may frequently be related to emotional stress and trauma. Releasing these bodily tensions may lead to emotional release and relaxation.

Self-Compassion: Yoga develops self-compassion and self-acceptance. Through the practice of non-judgmental awareness and self-care, people may establish a stronger connection with themselves, supporting emotional well-being.

Neuroplasticity: Regular yoga practice has been found to improve neuroplasticity, the brain's capacity to change and reorganize itself. This may lead to improved emotional reactions and greater emotional resilience over time.

Community and Support: Participating in group yoga sessions or practicing yoga in a community context may give a feeling of belonging and social support, which are key components in sustaining mental well-being.

Self-Reflection: The contemplative features of yoga give chances for self-reflection and introspection. This self-inquiry may lead to better self-awareness, enhanced emotional control, and personal development.

It's crucial to emphasize that although yoga may be tremendously good for mental well-being, it might not be a solo answer for everyone. It may be particularly useful when paired with other types of treatment, such as counseling or psychotherapy, for persons coping with more complicated emotional difficulties.

Incorporating yoga into your practice for emotional balance should be addressed with consistency and care. Finding the perfect type of yoga, teacher, and degree of practice that resonates with you may make a major difference in getting the intended emotional benefits. Always contact a healthcare practitioner before beginning a new exercise or fitness plan, particularly if you have pre-existing physical or mental health concerns.

Nourishing the Body with Fertility-Boosting Nutrition

Nourishing the body with a fertility-boosting diet is a matter of considerable relevance for people and couples who are attempting to conceive. Diet plays a critical part in optimizing fertility, as specific nutrients and dietary patterns may favorably improve reproductive health in both men and women. Here, we'll address crucial components of a fertility-boosting diet for both genders:

For Women:

Balanced Diet: Eating a balanced diet that includes a range of nutrient-rich foods is necessary. Focus on nutritious grains, lean meats, healthy fats, and a colorful variety of fruits and vegetables.

Folate: Adequate folate consumption is vital for avoiding birth abnormalities and sustaining early pregnancy. Leafy greens, lentils, beans, and fortified grains are rich sources of folate.

Iron: Iron is vital for sustaining good ovulation and supporting the increased blood volume during pregnancy. Include lean red meats, poultry, fish, legumes, and fortified grains.

Omega-3 Fatty Acids: Found in fatty fish (like salmon and sardines), flaxseeds, and walnuts, omega-3 fatty acids may help balance hormones and promote the general function of reproductive organs.

Antioxidants: Vitamins C and E, selenium, and beta-carotene are antioxidants that may help preserve eggs from harm and increase egg quality. Excellent sources include berries, citrus fruits, nuts, and seeds.

Dairy or Calcium Alternatives: Adequate calcium consumption is crucial for bone health. Opt for low-fat dairy products or fortified plant-based milk substitutes.

Healthy Weight: Maintaining a healthy weight is vital for hormonal balance and ovulation. Both being underweight and overweight might influence fertility.

For Men:

Zinc: Zinc is vital for sperm production and quality. Oysters, lean meats, nuts, and seeds are rich sources of zinc.

Selenium: This mineral helps prevent sperm from oxidative damage and promotes healthy sperm production. Include Brazil nuts, lean meats, and shellfish.

Vitamin D: Vitamin D is connected to testosterone levels and sperm quality. Spend time in the sun and incorporate fatty fish, fortified dairy products, and egg yolks into your diet.

Antioxidants: Just like in women, antioxidants are vital for male fertility too. Vitamins C and E, as well as selenium and coenzyme Q10, may all have good benefits on sperm quality.

Omega-3 Fatty Acids: Omega-3s help to good sperm membrane function. Fatty salmon, flaxseeds, and chia seeds are excellent sources.

Lycopene: Found in tomatoes and watermelon, lycopene is connected with enhanced sperm quality.

Limit Processed Foods and Trans Fats: Diets heavy in processed foods and trans fats may lead to inflammation and significantly damage sperm quality.

In addition to concentrating on certain nutrients, keeping a healthy lifestyle is vital. This includes controlling stress, getting regular exercise, keeping hydrated, and avoiding excessive alcohol and caffeine usage. For both spouses, avoiding smoking and recreational drugs is vital, since they may drastically decrease fertility. Remember, fertility is a complicated problem, and diet is only one component of the jigsaw. If you're dealing with fertility, it's crucial to speak with a healthcare expert or a fertility specialist to treat any underlying medical concerns and get individualized counsel.

Chapter 4: Yoga Practices for Fertility Enhancement

Yoga is typically considered a holistic approach to promoting overall well thought to boost fertility and reproductive health. While yoga alone may not ensure fertility enhancement, it can help decrease stress, regulate hormones, and increase blood circulation, which are aspects that might favorably affect fertility. **Here are some yoga postures that are typically advised for fertility enhancement:**

Deep Breathing and Meditation: Deep breathing practices, such as pranayama, assist in relieving tension and promote relaxation. Stress may have a detrimental influence on fertility, thus practicing mindfulness meditation and deep breathing might be useful.

Supta Baddha Konasana (Reclining Bound Angle Pose): This position opens the hips and groin regions, helping to enhance blood flow to the pelvic region. It's supposed to stimulate the ovaries and uterus.

Viparita Karani (Legs-Up-The-Wall Pose): This moderate inversion improves blood flow to the pelvic region and may help relieve tension. It's commonly performed to promote reproductive health.

Bharadvaja's Twist: This sitting twist may aid digestion and activate the abdominal organs, especially the reproductive functions. It's a terrific position for general pelvic wellness.

Bhramari Pranayama (Humming Bee Breath): This pranayama practice may have a relaxing impact on the nervous system, lowering tension and anxiety. It's also considered to activate the thyroid gland, which plays a role in regulating hormones.

Uttanasana (Standing Forward Bend): This forward fold helps stretch the back muscles and enhance blood circulation to the pelvic region.

Adho Mukha Svanasana (Downward-Facing Dog Pose): This position increases blood circulation to the pelvic area and stretches the back and hamstrings.

Agnisaar Kriya: This cleaning method includes fast abdominal contractions and releases. It's supposed to stimulate the digestive tract and help regulate hormones.

Yoni Mudra: A symbolic hand motion that concentrates energy on the pelvic region, fostering a connection with the reproductive organs.

Balasana (Child's Pose): This resting position may help alleviate tension in the back and promote relaxation.

Savasana (Corpse Pose): This last relaxation posture helps the body and mind to relax fully, which may help decrease stress and increase general well-being.

Remember that every person is unique, so it's vital to check with a healthcare expert before beginning any new workout or yoga practice, particularly if you have any underlying health concerns. While yoga may be a beneficial complement to a fertility-enhancing strategy, it's only one component, and maintaining a balanced lifestyle that includes a good diet, frequent exercise, and stress management is vital for fertility improvement.

Gentle Asanas to Regulate Hormones

Gentle asanas, or yoga positions, maybe a good approach to manage hormones in the body. Hormones serve a key role in sustaining numerous biological processes, including metabolism, mood, sleep, and general well-being. Engaging in a regular mild yoga practice may help balance hormones, decrease stress, and boost general wellness. Here are some mild asanas that are known to have a favorable influence on hormone regulation:

Child's Pose (Balasana): This soothing position helps relax the nervous system and decrease stress, which may lead to hormone imbalances. It also extends the lower back and hips, which helps ease stress and stiffness.

Cat-Cow Pose (Marjaryasana-Bitilasana): This dynamic combination of postures serves to gently massage the spine, stimulate the digestive system, and maintain a healthy balance in the endocrine system.

Downward-Facing Dog (Adho Mukha Svanasana): This position helps enhance blood circulation and may activate the thyroid gland, which is vital for controlling metabolism and energy levels.

Bridge Pose (Setu Bandhasana): By expanding the chest and lengthening the spine, Bridge Pose may help ease tension and anxiety. It also stimulates the thyroid gland and may assist in controlling hormonal functioning.

Supported Reclining Bound Angle Pose (Supta Baddha Konasana): This restorative posture helps expand the hips and gently stretches the groin region. It may stimulate the reproductive organs and enhance hormonal balance.

Legs-Up-the-Wall Pose (Viparita Karani): This inversion stance helps enhance blood circulation and may have a relaxing impact on the nervous system. It also supports the thyroid and parathyroid glands.

Seated Forward Bend (Paschimottanasana): This position may help decrease tension and promote digestion. It softly massages the stomach organs and helps enhance hormonal balance.

Corpse Pose (Savasana): This relaxation stance is vital for enabling the body to recuperate and regenerate. It may help decrease stress, increase sleep quality, and support overall hormonal balance.

Cobra Pose (Bhujangasana): This simple backbend may activate the adrenal glands, helping to control stress chemicals like cortisol. It also expands the chest and improves posture.

Easy Pose (Sukhasana) with Forward Fold: Sitting in a comfortable cross-legged posture and softly folding forward may help quiet the mind and decrease tension. This, in turn, fosters optimal hormonal balance.

When practicing these asanas, it's vital to concentrate on your breath and listen to your body. Avoid forcing oneself into postures that create pain or discomfort. A continuous mild yoga practice, along with a healthy lifestyle, good diet, and sufficient sleep, may have a significant influence on hormone control and general well-being.

However, if you have certain hormonal imbalances or medical concerns, it's essential to contact a healthcare practitioner before beginning any new exercise plan, including yoga. They may give individualized assistance based on your unique requirements and circumstances.

Surya Namaskar (Sun Salutations) Variation

Gentle asanas, or yoga positions, maybe a good approach to manage hormones in the body. Hormones serve a key role in sustaining numerous biological processes, including metabolism, mood, sleep, and general well-being. Engaging in a regular mild yoga practice may help balance hormones, decrease stress, and boost general wellness. Here are some mild asanas that are known to have a favorable influence on hormone regulation:

Child's Pose (Balasana): This soothing position helps relax the nervous system and decrease stress, which may lead to hormone imbalances. It also extends the lower back and hips, which helps ease stress and stiffness.

Cat-Cow Pose (Marjaryasana-Bitilasana): This dynamic combination of postures serves to gently massage the spine, stimulate the digestive system, and maintain a healthy balance in the endocrine system.

Downward-Facing Dog (Adho Mukha Svanasana): This position helps enhance blood circulation and may activate the thyroid gland, which is vital for controlling metabolism and energy levels.

Bridge Pose (Setu Bandhasana): By expanding the chest and lengthening the spine, Bridge Pose may help ease tension and anxiety. It also stimulates the thyroid gland and may assist in controlling hormonal functioning.

Supported Reclining Bound Angle Pose (Supta Baddha Konasana): This restorative posture helps expand the hips and gently stretches the groin region. It may stimulate the reproductive organs and enhance hormonal balance.

Legs-Up-the-Wall Pose (Viparita Karani): This inversion stance helps enhance blood circulation and may have a relaxing impact on the nervous system. It also supports the thyroid and parathyroid glands.

Seated Forward Bend (Paschimottanasana): This position

may help decrease tension and promote digestion. It softly massages the stomach organs and helps enhance hormonal balance.

Corpse Pose (Savasana): This relaxation stance is vital for enabling the body to recuperate and regenerate. It may help decrease stress, increase sleep quality, and support overall hormonal balance.

Cobra Pose (Bhujangasana): This simple backbend may activate the adrenal glands, helping to control stress chemicals like cortisol. It also expands the chest and improves posture.

Easy Pose (Sukhasana) with Forward Fold: Sitting in a comfortable cross-legged posture and softly folding forward may help quiet the mind and decrease tension. This, in turn, fosters optimal hormonal balance.

When practicing these asanas, it's vital to concentrate on your breath and listen to your body. Avoid forcing oneself into postures that create pain or discomfort. A continuous mild yoga practice, along with a healthy lifestyle, good diet, and sufficient sleep, may have a significant influence on hormone control and general well-being.

However, if you have certain hormonal imbalances or medical concerns, it's essential to contact a healthcare practitioner before beginning any new exercise plan, including yoga. They may give individualized assistance based on your unique requirements and circumstances.

Butterfly Pose (Baddha Konasana)

Butterfly position, also known as Baddha Konasana, is a yoga asana (position) that delivers several advantages for the body and mind. This stance is called by the way the legs and feet mimic the wings of a butterfly. It is a sitting position that includes bringing the feet together and letting the knees slide outwards, imitating the opening and shutting of butterfly wings. Here's a debate about the pose:

How to Practice Butterfly Pose:

Sit down on the floor with your legs out in front of you to begin.

Bend your knees and bring the soles of your feet together, allowing your knees to sink outwards.

Hold onto your feet or ankles with your hands, generating moderate pressure to urge your knees closer to the ground.

Sit up tall, elongating your spine.

You may gently flap your knees up and down, imitating the movement of a butterfly's wings. This might assist in alleviating tension in the hips.

Breathe deeply and keep the stance for a particular length, as comfortable.

Benefits of Butterfly Pose:

Hip Opening: Butterfly Pose is recognized for its ability to open up the hips and groin region. It stretches the inner thighs, hip flexors, and groin muscles, helping to enhance flexibility and mobility in the hip joints.

Improved Circulation: The position improves blood flow to the pelvic region, which may have favorable benefits on reproductive organs and general pelvic health.

Relaxation: Butterfly position is commonly used as a relaxing position or during meditation. The moderate flapping of the knees may generate a calming pattern that benefits relaxation and stress reduction.

Preparation for Childbirth: This position is occasionally suggested for pregnant women since it might assist in expanding the pelvis and ease strain on the lower back. It may also assist in childbirth preparation.

Digestive Benefits: Butterfly Pose may activate the abdominal organs, particularly the digestive system, which can aid in improving digestion and ease digestive pain.

Energy Flow: In yoga philosophy, the hips are considered a place of stagnated energy. Practicing Butterfly Pose may help release and circulate this energy.

Stretching the Groin and Thighs: The posture delivers a deep stretch to the inner thighs and groin region, which may be especially good for persons who spend a lot of time sitting or have tight hips.

Precautions:

Knee Sensitivity: If you have knee ailments or pain, be careful when performing this position. Place a blanket or pillow beneath your knees for support.

Flexibility: If your hips are stiff, you may not be able to bring your knees to the ground. Don't push the movement; allow your body to gently expand out over time.

Back Issues: If you have lower back difficulties, perform this position with care. Sit on a pillow or blanket to raise your hips slightly and lessen tension on the lower back.

Modifications: You may use props like cushions or blocks beneath your knees to make the posture more accessible and comfortable.

As with every yoga posture, it's crucial to listen to your body and practice with awareness. If you're new to yoga or have any health issues, it's a good idea to visit a competent yoga teacher or healthcare practitioner before trying new positions.

Supported Bridge Pose (Setu Bandhasana)

Supported Bridge Pose, also known as Setu Bandhasana, is a popular yoga asana that provides several physical and mental advantages. It falls to the group of backbends and is considered a benign inversion position. This position includes laying on your back and elevating your hips off the ground, creating a bridge-like configuration with your body. "Setu Bandhasana" originates from the Sanskrit words "setu," meaning "bridge," "bandha," meaning "lock" or "bind," and "asana," meaning "pose."

Here's how to practice Supported Bridge Pose (Setu Bandhasana):

Instructions:

Preparation: Begin by laying flat on your back with your knees bent and feet hip-width apart. Your feet should be situated near enough to your hips so you can touch your heels with your fingers.

Positioning: Press your feet and arms against the floor. Inhale, then as you exhale, gently raise your hips off the ground, using your glutes and core muscles. Keep your arms across your body with your hands facing down.

Rolling the Shoulders: Roll your shoulders beneath you, interlacing your fingers together. This movement will assist in elevating your chest slightly and generate room in your throat and neck.

Lift and Open: Continue to push down with your feet and shoulders as you raise your hips higher. Keep your thighs parallel to each other. Make sure your weight is equally distributed over your feet, shoulders, and arms.

Relax the Neck and Jaw: Relax your neck and let your head rest on the ground. Ensure your neck is comfortable and free from stress.

Breathing: Breathe deeply and evenly in this stance. You may also try taking deep breaths into your chest and belly to expand the chest and assist in opening through the front of the body.

Hold and Release: Hold the stance for several breaths or as long as feels comfortable. To release, breathe, and carefully drop your hips back to the ground, vertebra by vertebra.

Benefits:

Stretching the Chest and Shoulders: Supported Bridge Pose serves to expand and stretch the chest, shoulders, and the front of the body, counteracting the effects of hunching over or sitting for lengthy durations.

Strengthening the Glutes and Core: The position activates and develops the glutes and core muscles, helping to enhance posture and support the spine.

Calming the Mind: The moderate inversion caused by this position may have a relaxing impact on the nervous system, lowering tension and anxiety.

Improving Digestion: The position may assist in accelerating digestion and easing stomach pain.

Relieving Back Pain: Supported Bridge Pose may give relief for moderate backaches and assist in reducing tension in the lower back.

Therapeutic Benefits: This stance may be helpful for patients with asthma, high blood pressure, and sleeplessness. It may also help reduce symptoms of menopause.

Modifications:

For individuals who may find the stance problematic, there are many adjustments available:

Use Props: Place a yoga block beneath your sacrum for support, enabling you to relax into the posture without straining.

Hip Distance Feet: Instead of moving your feet close to your hips, consider positioning your feet hip-width apart to generate additional stability.

Shoulder Position: If interlacing your fingers below you is unpleasant, just lay your arms beside your body with your palms facing down.

As with any yoga posture, it's vital to practice mindfulness and listen to your body. If you have any pre-existing medical concerns or injuries, it's essential to visit a skilled yoga teacher or healthcare expert before trying Supported Bridge Pose or any other new practice.

Pranayama Techniques for Hormonal Balance

Pranayama, a practice of breath control in yoga, has been related to several health benefits, including supporting hormonal balance. Hormones have a critical role in controlling different biological processes, from metabolism to mood, and pranayama practices are thought to impact the endocrine system, which creates and controls hormones. **Here are some pranayama methods that are commonly advised to assist in achieving hormonal balance:**

Anulom Vilom (Alternate Nostril Breathing): This method includes exchanging the breath between the left and right nostrils. It is supposed to regulate the energy flow in the body and activate the pineal gland, which is responsible for creating melatonin and regulating sleep cycles. A balanced pineal gland might contribute to overall hormonal stability.

Bhramari (Humming Bee Breath): Bhramari entails creating a humming sound while exhaling slowly. This exercise is said to have a relaxing impact on the nervous system and activate the thyroid gland. The thyroid gland generates hormones that control metabolism and energy levels.

Sheetali (Cooling Breath): Sheetali includes breathing via a rolled tongue or slightly open lips and expelling through the nose. This approach is thought to chill the body and mind, perhaps assisting in lowering stress chemicals like cortisol.

Ujjayi (Victorious Breath): Ujjayi entails inhaling deeply and smoothly via the nose while gently tightening the back of the throat, generating a pleasant ocean-like sound. This approach may have a relaxing impact and assist in regulating the adrenal glands, which generate stress chemicals.

Kapalabhati (Skull Shining Breath): Kapalabhati is a strong exhalation method followed by passive inhalations.

It is supposed to purify the body and activate the abdominal organs, especially

the pancreas and adrenal glands, which play a role in hormone balance.

Sitali (Cooling Breath): Similar to Sheetali, Sitali includes breathing via a curled tongue or open mouth. It is supposed to provide a cooling and relaxing impact on the body and mind, perhaps helping to regulate stress-related chemicals.

Bhastrika (Bellows Breath): Bhastrika includes quick and strong inhalations and exhalations. This dynamic approach may stimulate the endocrine system and enhance oxygen delivery to the body's cells, thereby aiding hormonal equilibrium.

It's crucial to note that although certain pranayama practices have been connected with possible advantages for hormone balance, scientific study in this area is sparse, and outcomes might vary from person to person. If you're interested in adding pranayama into your practice for hormonal balance or any other health purpose, it's suggested to learn from a skilled yoga teacher and check with a healthcare practitioner, particularly if you have any underlying health concerns. Pranayama should support a comprehensive approach to health, including good diet, exercise, and stress management.

Bhramari Pranayama (Humming Bee Breath)

Bhramari Pranayama, sometimes referred to as Humming Bee Breath, is a breathing method originating from the ancient practice of Pranayama in Yoga. It includes making a humming sound while exhaling, which is said to offer many physical, mental, and spiritual advantages. This technique is called after the black Indian bee, Bhramari, because of the humming sound that is evocative of the bee's buzz. Bhramari Pranayama is regarded as a peaceful and meditative method that may aid in lowering stress, and anxiety, and increasing general well-being.

Here's how Bhramari Pranayama is commonly practiced:

Preparation:

Sit in a comfortable and peaceful spot with your back straight and shoulders relaxed. You may sit in a cross-legged posture on the floor or a chair with your feet flat on the ground. Begin by sitting on the floor, legs outstretched in front of you.

Hand Placement: Place your index fingers on your ears, softly pushing the tragus (the little pointed cartilage on the outer ear canal) to block up the ear canal. This will help shut out extraneous noises.

Inhale: Take a slow and deep breath through your nose, filling your lungs with air.

Exhale with Humming:

As you exhale, softly press your fingers on the tragus to partly seal your ears and produce gentle pressure. While exhaling, generate a humming sound akin to the buzzing of a bee. The sound should be quiet and resonant, emanating from the back of your throat. Keep the music steady throughout the exhale, allowing it to echo throughout your brain.

Breath Retention (Optional):

After exhaling, you may hold your breath for a second while keeping your eyes closed and concentrating on the feelings inside. Then, remove the fingers from your ears and inhale slowly and deeply through your nose.

Repeat: Repeat this practice for numerous rounds, striving to maintain the breath calm, smooth, and relaxed. You may practice Bhramari Pranayama for a few minutes to start and progressively extend the time as you grow more familiar with the method.

The advantages claimed to Bhramari Pranayama include:

Stress Reduction: The quiet humming sound and regulated breath may have a relaxing impact on the neurological system, helping to ease stress, anxiety, and tension.

Relaxation: The technique induces a state of relaxation by stimulating the parasympathetic nervous system, which is responsible for the "rest and digest" response.

Improved Concentration: Regular practice of Bhramari Pranayama is considered to promote attention and concentration.

Alleviation of Anger and Frustration: The relaxing aspect of the practice might assist in regulating emotions like anger and irritation.

Throat Health: The vibrations released during the humming sound might have good benefits on the throat and voice chords.

Spiritual Connection: Some practitioners think that Bhramari Pranayama helps promote a sense of inner serenity and connection with the self.

As with any yoga practice, it's crucial to listen to your body and not push any element of the practice. If you encounter pain or dizziness, you should stop the practice and see a healthcare practitioner or a competent yoga teacher before resuming.

Nadi Shodhana Pranayama (Alternate Nostril Breathing)

Which is also known as Alternate Nostril Breathing, is a strong and popular breathing method in the practice of yoga and meditation. It comprises rhythmic and regulated breathing via alternating nostrils, with the purpose of harmonizing the body's energy pathways (nadis) and soothing the mind. The term "Nadi" alludes to the subtle energy pathways in the body, while "Shodhana" implies purification or cleaning. Therefore, Nadi Shodhana Pranayama might be interpreted as "Purifying Breath for Energy Channels."

Technique:

Preparation: Find a comfortable seating posture. You may employ the traditional position like Padmasana (Lotus Pose) or just sit cross-legged. Make sure your spine is straight and your hands are resting on your knees with palms facing up.

Hand Position (Mudra): Use your right thumb to seal your right nostril and your right ring finger to close your left nostril.

Breathing Pattern: Close your right nostril with your right thumb and inhale deeply and slowly through your left nostril.

Once you've breathed entirely, shut your left nostril with your right ring finger and release your right nose.

Exhale gently and fully via your right nostril.

Inhale deeply and gently via your right nostril.

Close your right nose again and release your left nostril.

Exhale gently and fully via your left nostril.

Repeat: Continue this alternate pattern for numerous rounds. Each cycle comprises one full intake and exhale via both nostrils.

Breath Awareness: As you practice, concentrate your attention on the breath, monitoring the feeling of the air passing through each nostril and the movement of your belly and chest.

Benefits:

Balances Energy: Nadi Shodhana is thought to balance the flow of prana (life force energy) in the body. The left nostril is related with the cooling, soothing, and receptive qualities, whereas the right nostril is associated with the heating, energizing, and active aspects. Alternate nostril breathing seeks to equalize these energies.

Calms the Mind: This pranayama method has a relaxing impact on the nerve system, helping to relieve tension, anxiety, and mental unrest. It increases mental clarity and concentrate.

Purification: The technique is claimed to cleanse the subtle energy pathways (nadis) in the body, clearing obstructions and facilitating smoother energy flow.

Enhances Respiratory Function: Nadi Shodhana stimulates slow, deep, and regulated breathing, which helps enhance lung capacity and oxygen exchange.

Stress Relief: By controlling the breath and concentrating the mind, this method generates a state of relaxation and may be a helpful tool for managing stress and emotional swings.

Precautions:

Start Slowly: If you're new to pranayama, begin with a few rounds and progressively increase the time as you grow more comfortable.

Avoid Strain: Keep your breath smooth and pleasant. Don't push or stretch the breath.

Consult a Professional: If you have any respiratory concerns or medical illnesses, see a healthcare expert or qualified yoga teacher before doing Nadi Shodhana.

Nadi Shodhana Pranayama is a flexible technique that may be included into your everyday yoga and meditation practice. It's a subtle but effective technique to balance your energy, quiet your mind, and boost your entire feeling of well-being.

Stress-Reducing Yoga Nidra for Relaxation

Yoga Nidra is a strong relaxation and meditation practice that attempts to produce profound relaxation and ease stress. It's commonly referred to as "yogic sleep" or "psychic sleep" since it takes you into a stage between awake and sleep, when significant relaxation and renewal may occur. Here's a discussion on how Yoga Nidra might assist relieve stress and promote relaxation:

Understanding Yoga Nidra:

Yoga Nidra is a systematic practice that includes laying down in a comfortable posture while the practitioner is led through a sequence of instructions. These instructions often incorporate body awareness, breath awareness, visualization, and cognitive awareness of diverse experiences. The technique methodically moves your attention through various sections of the body, establishing a sensation of relaxation and letting go of physical and mental stress.

Stress Reduction with Yoga Nidra:

Deep Relaxation: Yoga Nidra generates a state of profound relaxation that helps soothe the nervous system. It changes the body from the "fight or flight" reaction (sympathetic nervous system) to the "rest and digest" mode (parasympathetic nervous system), which promotes relaxation and healing.

Reduction of Anxiety: By concentrating the mind on body sensations, breath, and imagination, Yoga Nidra may help deflect attention from stressful thoughts. It facilitates a change from brooding on the past or worrying about the future to being present in the now.

Release of Tensions: The exercise progressively walks you through various sections of the body, helping you to become aware of any physical tensions or discomforts. With this knowledge, you may intentionally release muscular tension and mental stress, encouraging physical and mental relaxation.

Improved Sleep Quality: Regular practice of Yoga Nidra might promote sleep quality. The practice's capacity to produce relaxation and settle the mind might aid people battling with insomnia or sleep difficulties.

Enhanced Mindfulness: Yoga Nidra cultivates awareness by directing your attention in a non-judgmental manner.

This mindfulness may extend into your everyday life, helping you react to challenges with better awareness and serenity.

Emotional Balance: The practice may bring awareness to emotions, helping you establish a healthy connection with them. By noticing feelings without getting overwhelmed by them, you may achieve emotional equilibrium.

Strengthened Resilience: With consistent practice, Yoga Nidra may enhance your ability to tolerate stress. It trains you to stay comfortable and composed even in tough conditions.

Practicing Yoga Nidra: To practice Yoga Nidra for stress reduction and relaxation:

Find a peaceful Space: Choose a peaceful and comfortable spot where you won't be interrupted.

Lie Down: Lie on your back in a comfortable posture, using cushions and blankets for comfort.

Follow Guidance: You may follow a guided Yoga Nidra session given by an instructor or utilize pre-recorded sessions.

Body Awareness: Follow the directions to become aware of various body parts and feelings.

Breath Awareness: Focus on your breath, observing its natural rhythm without attempting to manipulate it.

Visualization: Engage in guided imagery to produce a feeling of peace and tranquillity.

Profound Relaxation: Allow yourself to achieve a state of profound relaxation, letting go of bodily and mental stress.

Closing: Slowly bring your awareness back to your surroundings, softly moving your fingers and toes before opening your eyes.

Conclusion:

Yoga Nidra is an effective therapy for stress reduction and relaxation. Regular practice may lead to enhanced general well-being, increased resistance to stress, and a stronger feeling of serenity in everyday life. Whether you're new to relaxation methods or have expertise with meditation, Yoga Nidra provides a unique approach that may help you attain profound realms of relaxation and inner peace.

Cultivating Core Strength for Pelvic Health

Cultivating core strength is a vital element of sustaining pelvic health. The core refers to the collection of muscles that offer stability and support to the spine, pelvis, and torso. These muscles comprise not only the well-known abdominal muscles (rectus abdominis, transverse abdominis), but also the muscles of the lower back, hips, and pelvic floor. Pelvic health, on the other hand, refers to the healthy functioning of the pelvic organs and tissues, including the bladder, uterus (in females), rectum, and pelvic floor muscles.

Here's how increasing core strength adds to pelvic health:

Stability and Support: A strong core offers a sturdy platform for your spine and pelvis. This stability is necessary for healthy alignment and movement of your pelvic organs. When the core muscles are weak, it may lead to poor alignment of the pelvis and greater pressure on the pelvic organs, possibly leading to complications such as incontinence and pelvic organ prolapse.

Pelvic Floor Support: The pelvic floor muscles constitute the basis of the core. These muscles perform a key function in supporting the pelvic organs and preserving continence. A strong core helps the pelvic floor muscles work correctly. Conversely, a weak core may lead to an imbalance in the pelvic floor muscles, possibly leading to urine or fecal incontinence.

Good Body Mechanics: Core strength is crucial for maintaining good body mechanics throughout numerous tasks, such as lifting, bending, and twisting. When you activate your core muscles, you establish a sturdy and supportive foundation for these motions, lessening the tension in your pelvic region.

Posture Improvement: Core strength is intimately connected to proper posture. When your core muscles are strong, they help you maintain an upright posture, which in turn minimizes the probability of pelvic misalignment and associated disorders.

Prevention and Management of Pain: Core strength may aid in relieving lower back pain and pelvic discomfort. Weak core muscles may lead to incorrect movement patterns, creating tension in the lower back and pelvis. Strengthening the core may help distribute the weight more evenly and lessen the likelihood of soreness.

Enhanced Circulation: Engaging the core muscles may assist in boosting blood circulation in the pelvic area. Improved circulation is vital for maintaining healthy pelvic organs and avoiding disorders like pelvic congestion.

To build core strength for pelvic health:

Engage in Core Exercises: Incorporate workouts that target all elements of the core, including the abdominal muscles, lower back, hips, and pelvic floor. Planks, bridges, pelvic tilts, and deep breathing exercises are great alternatives.

Practice attentive Movement: Be attentive to your posture and movement throughout the day. Engage your core muscles while lifting items, sitting, standing, and walking.

Stay Active: Regular physical exercise, such as strength training, yoga, and Pilates, may help enhance core strength and general pelvic health.

Pelvic Floor Exercises: Consider doing pelvic floor exercises (Kegels) to particularly target the muscles that support the pelvic organs.

Consult Professionals: If you're new to exercising or have particular pelvic health problems, consider seeing a physical therapist or healthcare specialist. They can advise you in designing a safe and effective core-strengthening practice suited to your requirements.

Remember that improving core strength requires time and persistence. By implementing these activities into your routine, you may enhance pelvic health and lower the risk of linked illnesses.

Chapter 5: Designing a Personalized Yoga Practice and Lifestyle Plan

Designing a customized yoga practice and lifestyle plan entails building a customized approach to yoga and everyday living that matches with an individual's objectives, requirements, preferences, and physical skills. It goes beyond merely following a conventional yoga program and extends to incorporating yogic ideas into different parts of life. Here's a step-by-step instruction on how to build such a plan:

Assessment and Goal Setting: Begin by having a detailed chat with the person to establish their current health state, fitness level, and any pre-existing medical illnesses, injuries, or limits. Also, enquire about their objectives, whether they're seeking stress alleviation, flexibility, strength, weight control, or spiritual development.

Customized Yoga Practice: Based on the evaluation, develop a yoga sequence that incorporates asanas (physical postures), pranayama (breathing exercises), and meditation techniques. Tailor the sequence to the individual's requirements, ensuring that it meets their objectives and acknowledges any physical constraints. Gradually develop the exercise to minimize boredom and foster growth.

Adaptation and Modification: Be prepared to change stances and approaches as required. Offer options for persons who may have injuries, medical concerns, or restricted mobility. The practice must be safe and sustainable for the person's circumstances.

Frequency and length: Determine the appropriate frequency and length of the yoga practice. This might range from a daily practice to many times a week, depending on the person's schedule, objectives, and physical condition.

Incorporating Yogic concepts: Encourage the integration of yogic concepts beyond the mat. This involves

161

practicing mindfulness, gratitude, self-awareness, and conscious breathing throughout the day. These concepts may help develop a healthy and peaceful living.

Nutrition and Hydration: Offer suggestions on a diet that compliments the yoga practice. Emphasize healthy, nutrient-rich meals and sufficient hydration. Tailor dietary suggestions depending on any particular health objectives, such as weight control or energy improvement.

Sleep and Rest: Highlight the significance of a regular sleep pattern and excellent slumber. Adequate sleep improves the body's healing and general well-being.

Stress Management: Provide practices for stress reduction, such as mindfulness meditation, relaxation exercises, and pranayama. Assist the person in understanding stress causes and establishing coping techniques.

Regular Check-ins and Adjustments: Schedule frequent check-ins to review progress, make appropriate modifications to the practice, and address any issues or concerns. Flexibility is crucial; the plan should adapt as the individual's requirements change.

Holistic Approach: Encourage a holistic approach to health by including additional activities that complement the yoga practice, such as walking, swimming, or other types of exercise. Also, try combining hobbies, social activities, and relaxing methods.

Mindful Self-Care: Teach the significancc of self-care and self-compassion. This involves setting aside time for oneself, participating in things that offer delight, and keeping a positive self-dialogue.

Long-Term Sustainability: Create a strategy that is long-term sustainable. Avoid severe activities that might lead to exhaustion or injury. The objective is to build a balanced, lifelong approach to yoga and well-being.

Remember, every individual is unique, and a tailored yoga practice and lifestyle plan should match their specific requirements and ambitions. Regular communication, flexibility, and a caring attitude are important for effective implementation. If you're not a trained yoga teacher or healthcare professional, consider incorporating such specialists in the creation and monitoring of the strategy.

Consulting with a Yoga Instructor and Medical Professional

Yoga teachers and medical professional consultations may provide a comprehensive approach to health and well-being that combines the advantages of physical exercise, mental calm, and medical knowledge. Let's look at how these two viewpoints can work together:

A yoga teacher:

A yoga teacher has received training to lead people through a variety of yoga practices with an emphasis on asanas (physical postures), pranayama (breathing exercises), meditation, and awareness. Having a conversation with a yoga teacher may have several advantages:

Physical Well-Being: Yoga may enhance one's balance, flexibility, strength, and posture. Yoga instructors may modify poses to suit certain physical restrictions or demands, such as back discomfort, joint problems, or tight muscles.

Stress management In yoga, relaxation and awareness are prioritized. Deep breathing and meditation are two practices that may ease anxiety and tension while also enhancing sleep.

Mental-Physical Connection: Mind-body awareness is fostered via yoga. Better body awareness and sensitivity to how physical activity or stresses affect general health might be encouraged by it.

Holistic strategy: Yoga aims to promote not just physical fitness but also mental, emotional, and spiritual health. A teacher can help people discover inner harmony and balance.

Medical Specialist:

A doctor or physical therapist, for example, contributes a scientific and medical viewpoint to the discussion. **Having a medical professional's advice has several significant benefits:**

Health Assessment: Medical experts may assess your current state of health, medical history, and any ailments you may already have. This knowledge is essential for choosing the kinds of physical activities that are healthy and helpful for you.

Prevention of Injuries: In particular, if you have any physical limits or pre-existing diseases, medical specialists may provide advice on how to avoid injury. They may provide suggestions for adjusting your yoga routine to suit your requirements.

Medically informed practices include: A medical expert may suggest certain yoga postures and practices that aid in your recovery whether you're recuperating from an accident or managing chronic health problems.

Personal recommendations include: If required, medical specialists may assist in creating a comprehensive health plan that incorporates yoga in addition to other medical treatments like drugs or physical therapy.

The combination of:

A medical practitioner and a yoga teacher working together may be very effective.

Complete Care: You gain from a balanced strategy that takes care of both your physical and medical requirements. If you have any unique health issues or restrictions, this is very crucial.

Safety First: Medical experts make sure that any yoga activities you engage in are suitable for your health situation, lowering the danger of worsening medical conditions.

Best Case Scenario: By focusing on both the physical and medicinal aspects of well-being, yoga poses suggested by both experts may enhance benefits.

Essentially, working with a yoga teacher and a medical specialist results in a complete approach to health that combines physical activity, mental well-being, and medical knowledge. This teamwork may result in better overall health, more energy, and a higher standard of living. Always bear in mind, to be honest with both experts and to advise them of any changes to your health.

Creating a Tailored Yoga Routine

Designing a series of yoga postures and practices that are customized to a person's requirements, objectives, and skills constitutes creating a personalized yoga program. As it targets your particular needs, a customized yoga regimen may be more successful and pleasurable than adhering to a generic plan.

The following is a step-by-step tutorial on how to design a customized yoga routine:

Determine Your Needs and Goals:

Choose a motivation for practicing yoga. Is it for stress reduction, relaxation, flexibility, strength, or something else?

Recognize any particular body parts that need care, such as your back, hips, or weak core muscles.

Take into account your level of fitness right now and any potential medical issues. If necessary, get advice from a medical expert.

Select the Different Yoga Styles: Yoga comes in a variety of forms with distinct advantages. For instance, Vinyasa yoga is more energetic and incorporates flowing sequences, while Hatha yoga emphasizes alignment and is perfect for beginners.

Pick a style that complements your interests and ambitions. To create a well-rounded workout, you could also mix several styles.

Select positions:

Do your homework and choose yoga positions that cater to your particular requirements and objectives. For instance, use postures that stretch the main muscle groups if you want to increase your flexibility.

Incorporate positions that target various body areas. A well-rounded exercise program should focus on balance, flexibility, strength, and relaxation.

Sequence the positions. Arrange the chosen poses in a sensible order. A program often begins with a warm-up, continues with increasingly challenging postures, and then cools down and relaxes.

As you go from simpler poses to more difficult ones, think about establishing a seamless, natural flow.

Consider pranayama (breath control) and meditation as part of your practice.

Consider Breathing and Meditation. These techniques improve relaxation and awareness.

Depending on your objectives, breathing exercises may be utilized to either invigorate or soothe the body.

Be Mindful of Alignment: To avoid injuries, pay close attention to each pose's correct alignment. Over time, improper alignment may cause strain or pain.

Consider attending a few yoga courses with a certified teacher if you're new to the practice to get the fundamentals of alignment.

Listen to Your Body: Never practice outside of your comfort zone and abstain from overexerting yourself. While challenging oneself shouldn't hurt, it is still vital.

Adjust positions as necessary. Yoga bolsters, blocks, and straps may help you ease into postures and achieve proper alignment.

Set a Realistic Schedule: Choose how often you'll use your customized routine. Select a frequency that fits with your schedule and responsibilities since consistency is important.

Monitor Your Progress: Maintain a diary to keep tabs on your development. Keep track of any changes in your strength, flexibility, or emotional and mental state.

Reassess and Adjust: Update your regimen as necessary as you advance and your requirements change. An early regimen that worked well can need adjustments over time.

Always keep in mind that developing a customized yoga program is a dynamic process. It ought to change to meet your evolving demands and goals. Consider consulting with a licensed yoga teacher or therapist for advice if you're hesitant about creating a practice on your own.

They may provide tailored suggestions based on your objectives and restrictions.

Integrating Yoga with Other Fertility Enhancement Strategies

Integrating yoga with other fertility enhancement treatments might be a comprehensive way to help people or couples who are trying to conceive. Fertility may be impacted by several variables, including stress, hormone balance, circulation, and general well-being. Yoga, with its emphasis on physical postures, breath control, meditation, and relaxation, might complement other fertility enhancement treatments by addressing these aspects.

Here's a discussion on how yoga may be incorporated with different approaches:

Stress Reduction: Stress may have a detrimental influence on fertility by changing hormone levels and the reproductive system. Yoga's focus on relaxation, deep breathing, and meditation may help relieve tension and develop a feeling of tranquility. Integrating yoga techniques like gentle postures (asanas) and mindfulness meditation might help with stress reduction, boosting the efficiency of reproductive therapies.

Hormonal Balance: Certain yoga positions are considered to activate the endocrine system, which plays a vital role in regulating hormones associated with conception. Poses that include moderate twists and inversions may enhance blood flow to the reproductive organs and help regulate hormones. Combining these postures with hormone-regulating diets and activities prescribed by medical practitioners may be useful.

Blood Circulation: Healthy blood circulation is crucial for the reproductive organs to operate efficiently. Yoga poses that include hip opening and pelvic floor engagement might enhance blood flow to the pelvic area, improving reproductive health. When coupled with activities such as regular exercise and dietary modifications, yoga may promote overall circulation.

Mind-Body Connection: Yoga lays major emphasis on the mind-body connection. Integrating yoga with other reproductive treatments encourages people to gain a greater awareness of their bodies and emotions. This self-awareness may help people recognize and manage any emotional or psychological concerns that could be impacting their reproductive journey.

Lifestyle and Diet: Integrating yoga with lifestyle modifications and a balanced diet may offer a holistic approach to fertility improvement. Yoga increases attentive eating and may promote better food choices.

Additionally, yoga may drive people to adopt a more active lifestyle, which can significantly improve fertility.

Partner Involvement: Fertility improvement is generally a collaborative journey for couples. Practicing yoga together may not only enhance physical health but also build an emotional tie between spouses. Partner yoga postures may be a pleasant and personal way to encourage each other on this journey.

Mindfulness and Acceptance: Fertility issues might lead to emotional pressure. Yoga's principles of mindfulness and acceptance may help folks deal with the uncertainties and emotional ups and downs of the reproductive process. This may be linked with therapy and support groups to produce a well-rounded strategy.

Personalized Approach: It's vital to realize that every individual's reproductive journey is unique. Integrating yoga with other fertility enhancement treatments should be personalized to the individual's requirements, medical recommendations, and preferences. Consulting with reproductive specialists, medical professionals, and experienced yoga teachers helps guarantee a safe and successful integration.

In conclusion, combining yoga with other reproductive enhancement treatments may provide a synergistic impact that addresses many physical, emotional, and psychological components of fertility. While yoga may be a beneficial tool, it should be considered as a complementary strategy alongside medical assistance and other evidence-based techniques.

Tracking Progress and Adapting Your Plan

Tracking progress and adjusting your plan are critical components of attaining personal and professional objectives, managing projects efficiently, and reacting to changes in varied circumstances. Whether you're an individual trying for personal growth or a team working on a difficult project, these methods may lead to improved results and higher success. Let's look into the necessity of measuring progress and changing plans, along with some techniques to execute them effectively:

Importance of Tracking Progress:

Visibility: Regularly monitoring progress offers a clear snapshot of where you are regarding your objectives. It helps you recognize successes, areas requiring development, and any possible impediments.

Motivation: Seeing visible improvement may raise motivation and sustain momentum. Celebrating minor triumphs along the road might motivate you to keep working towards your objectives.

Accountability: Tracking progress makes you responsible for your promises. When you have a record of your triumphs and failures, it's simpler to accept responsibility for your actions and choices.

Early Problem Identification: By monitoring your progress, you may spot concerns early on and take remedial steps before they grow into serious obstacles.

Flexibility: Tracking progress helps you to determine if your initial idea is functioning as planned. If not, you may make essential modifications without blindly clinging to a poor method.

Strategies for Tracking Progress:

Set Measurable Goals: Define clear, defined, and quantifiable objectives. This gives a framework for measuring your development objectively.

Use Key Performance Indicators (KPIs): KPIs are quantitative measurements that let you assess your development. They might be financial, operational, or performance-related, depending on the circumstances.

Regular Check-ins: Schedule frequent intervals to assess your progress. This might be daily, weekly, monthly, or project-specific. Use these check-ins to measure how far you've come and what needs change.

Visual Aids: Graphs, charts, and other visual aids may help you see your development over time. This makes trends and patterns more visible.

Document Your Journey: Keep a record of your triumphs, failures, and the activities you take to resolve obstacles. This paperwork may give insights into your decision-making process.

Adapting Your Plan:

Flexibility: While it's necessary to have a strategy, being excessively strict might inhibit growth. Embrace flexibility and be open to revising your strategy depending on new conditions.

Evaluate Effectiveness: Regularly examine if your existing strategy is helping you accomplish your objectives. If not, evaluate what adjustments are required.

Identify Roadblocks: When you meet hurdles, don't shy away from adjusting your strategy to solve them. Adaptation could require altering techniques, acquiring extra resources, or even rethinking your aims.

Feedback and Lessons Learned: Collect input from stakeholders, peers, or mentors. Their thoughts may shine light on blind areas and suggest essential adjustments.

Risk Management: Continuously examine possible hazards that might damage your strategy. Have contingency plans in place to manage these risks if they occur.

Prioritize: Not all changes or problems demand instant adaptation. Prioritize what requires attention based on effect and immediacy.

In summary, assessing progress and changing plans are dynamic processes that support success and development. They help people and teams to remain connected with their objectives while keeping sensitive to changes and difficulties. By adopting these techniques, you may handle uncertainty more successfully and make informed choices that lead to beneficial results.

Celebrating Self-Care and the Journey to Conception

The path to conception, distinguished by the desire to create or expand a family, is a major and intensely personal event for many people and couples. It includes a complex combination of physical, emotional, and psychological variables that may be both enjoyable and demanding. In recent years, there has been a rising focus on the necessity of self-care during this process, realizing that taking care of one's well-being is vital to navigating the ups and downs of trying to conceive.

Self-Care along the Journey to Conception:

Physical Health: Maintaining a healthy lifestyle is vital while trying to conceive. This involves eating a balanced diet, being active, and controlling any existing health concerns. Regular exercise and a balanced diet not only enhance fertility but also help general well-being.

Emotional Well-being: The emotional part of the road to conception is frequently neglected. The expectation, optimism, and occasionally disappointment may take a toll on mental health. Engaging in activities that relieve stress, such as meditation, yoga, writing, or spending quality time with loved ones, may help manage these feelings.

Communication: Open and honest communication with one's relationship is crucial. Both people may have diverse emotions and coping techniques. Creating a safe environment for dialogues about fears, expectations, and worries may enhance the relationship and give mutual support.

Support System: Building a support network is vital. This may include friends, relatives, or even support groups of individuals going through similar circumstances. Sharing one's sentiments with someone who understands may be very soothing.

Managing Expectations: While it's normal to be delighted and optimistic, it's also crucial to understand that the route to conception may be unexpected. Managing expectations and being prepared for future obstacles might help reduce excessive stress.

Seeking Professional Help: If the trip becomes extremely tough or extended, obtaining aid from medical specialists is encouraged. Fertility experts may give information, run required tests, and provide viable treatments.

Celebrating Self-Care:

Celebrating self-care on the path to conception is about acknowledging that taking care of oneself is not selfish, but rather a necessary part of the process. **Here are a few ideas for celebrating self-care:**

Milestone Recognition: Celebrate each stage of the road, whether it's a month of good behavior, a milestone in medical treatments, or a moment of emotional breakthrough. Acknowledging progress, no matter how modest, may bring encouragement and happiness.

Self-Compassion: Treat oneself with care and understanding. It's normal to experience a variety of emotions throughout this time, and practicing self-compassion enables self-acceptance without judgment.

Pampering Rituals: Engage in activities that offer delight and relaxation. This might be anything from having a bubble bath, indulging oneself in a spa day, or just taking a stroll in nature.

Connection with spouse: Plan frequent date nights or quality time with one's spouse. Focusing on the connection outside of the route to conception may help preserve a solid link.

Hobbies & Interests: Pursue activities and interests that provide enjoyment. Engaging in creative or rewarding hobbies may serve as a beneficial diversion and increase overall well-being.

In Conclusion:

The path to conception is a unique and momentous phase in many people's lives. Celebrating self-care on this journey is not just a method of sustaining one's well-being but also a chance to appreciate the perseverance, fortitude, and determination that the process demands. By emphasizing physical health, mental well-being, and strong relationships, individuals and couples may traverse this journey with grace, patience, and self-love.

Remember, each individual's journey is unique, and while yoga can be a valuable tool for enhancing fertility, it's important to consult with a healthcare provider before making significant lifestyle changes. This guide aims to provide a comprehensive overview of incorporating yoga into a fertility-focused approach after PCOS/PCOD, but personalized guidance is key to achieving the best results.